Breaking

LIMITS

Turning disability into possibility

Bart Gee

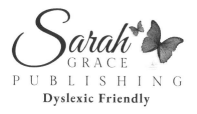

Sarah GRACE PUBLISHING
Dyslexic Friendly

First published 2019 by Sarah Grace Publishing an imprint of Malcolm Down
Publishing Ltd.
www.malcolmdown.co.uk

British Library Cataloguing in Publication Data
A catalogue record for this book is available from the British Library.

ISBN 978-1-912863-03-7

Cover photograph by Leanne Punshon at Little Bird Photography
Additional photography by Christian Television Association
Cover design by Esther Kotecha
Art direction by Sarah Grace

Printed in the UK

Contents

Foreword
by Bart's mum, Lynne

———

'It's a lovely boy,' were the words of the professor as he delivered my baby. 'What are you going to call him?'

'Bartholomew,' was my reply.

'And what is your other son called?'

'Samuel,' I replied

'Good Bible names,' was his reaction, and probably going through his mind was that I would need my Christian faith for what was to come.

Bartholomew was put into my arms and I felt the joy most mothers feel when they have their first cuddle.

'He is going to need some help,' was the next comment, but nothing would detract from those precious first moments.

The next day, so many white coats came to see me and to see Bartholomew that I realised that this was going to be much more of challenge than I had initially thought. It was really very traumatic with lots of different opinions and I remember picking him up from his cot and thinking, 'What have we done to produce this!' What kind of problems would this little boy have to face? Would he be an outcast? And the funniest thing – would anyone want to marry him?

Then, peace came from heaven and I felt overwhelmed in my little ward with the sense of the Lord's presence. I felt 'This little boy is our gift from God' and I remembered a verse I was asked to read way back in school assembly: 'If I ask Him for bread, will He give me a stone? If I ask him for fish, etc.' and I felt a strong conviction that everything would be alright.

The following evening I had just drifted off to sleep when I was awakened by a nurse who said that they had been observing for several hours and felt that Bart should go into special care, so would I get up and go with him? The two hours that followed were very difficult to handle as I was told that he was very ill, to expect the worst and anything else would be a bonus! In the early hours they asked if I would like to call my husband but I declined, thinking he needed to sleep if he was to face a big problem later. However, we were part of a lovely Christian fellowship and we had the backing of our church who prayed earnestly and I was told that one of our special friends who was normally fairly reserved, reached heaven. Heaven responded! And gradually my baby recovered.

The medical team didn't want me to leave hospital without Bartholomew but suggested that I started to make trips out with my husband, David, and Samuel. I had already been in hospital for two months so re-entry into normal life had to be gradual. The medical staff and everyone involved were so kind to me and if I went out in the evening, I would return to my room, lights being on and covers back, just as though I was in a lovely hotel. The nurses became my friends, always ready to listen and to encourage. I couldn't speak more highly of the treatment I received.

The first Sunday, Bart being tucked up in his cot in SCBU (Special Care Baby Unit), we paid our first visit to church and what a morning it was! This was to shape our whole future. You see, the Lord spoke through prophesy and said that little by little things would change and people were going to look and would be amazed... and what has happened? Exactly that!

After four weeks Bart was discharged. Carol, one of the Christian nurses, brought him to the car, said, 'I love you, Bartholomew' and placed him in the car and we said our goodbyes. We were bound for home and all that the future had to hold for the four of us.

I went home, leaving the security of the hospital, in the knowledge that I had a husband who loved me, a little boy who needed me, a church that would support me and a Saviour who knew every step that we would take. With this knowledge our new life was going to be a different experience.

The physio department became our second home. Three times a week I would sort the children, get them into the car and drive to Bristol children's hospital. Jane, our physio, an expert in her field, did everything to help us make our life as normal as possible and gave Bart the help that his body was crying out for. When I first met Jane I immediately had confidence in her ability and was convinced that if any human being could do something for him, she was just that person.

Our times in the physio department were not dull. I was shown how to do physio, Bart was stretched, pulled, plastered but most of all loved, while Samuel played and used the equipment as though he was at playschool. It was a very happy environment and of course we met countless numbers of children with difficulties and their families in the process.

At home, we lived as normally as we possibly could and adapted very quickly to our new life. The first Sunday after we came home, Bart was dedicated to the Lord and I remember standing, surrounded by our friends and church family, praying and just saying, 'Lord, he is Yours!' I believe our friends joined with us in submitting him to the Lord and it is obvious that the Lord's blessing has been upon his life. An elderly lady who had been a midwife said after the service, 'He'll be fine, he's got a fine pair of lungs!'

Our pastor prayed an inspired prayer – that we would see Bart walk down the aisle and that he would play the organ like his dad! At a very early age Bart's personality started to show and we could see that we had a determined, content and happy child, and our desire was that we would nurture this so that he would develop into as good an all-rounder as possible, always remembering the 'little by little'.

Bart had very little movement in his arms because of stiff joints and lack of muscles, but for the first Christmas (by now he was eight months old) we gave him a rainbow stacking frame, where the rings were put on in sequence. How was he going to do this? He worked and worked and worked at it. There was no giving up, such was his determination, and by the end of the day the stand was complete, giving us and him the joy of knowing that what looked impossible could be achieved. We experienced this so much, which always spurred us on to the next thing.

We always had lots of music in the home and as a very little baby, his love of music became apparent. I would place him on the floor and one leg would rock in time with music that Daddy would play on the piano, and this was the start of Bart's natural musical talent. Anything with which he could make sounds was a delight to him so we bought him his first xylophone, strapped the hammers to his hands and off he went – the start of a life enriched by music and the satisfaction that this gives.

Bart has had several major operations throughout his life. With the first one, as probably with all of them, I felt very apprehensive. We saw a house doctor who was checking him in who asked me how I was coping. Inside I thought, 'Not very well really' because I didn't find the operation scene easy at all, but went on to tell her that I was a Christian and how that sustained me – I said, 'I believed in divine strength!' I asked if she went to church and she said that she didn't but she had friends who were Christians. The next day she came into the ward and said she had had dinner the previous evening with friends who went to my church and they told her that everyone was praying for Bart. Subsequently her friends told me that they had been praying for her, that she would become a Christian and that my word was timely. I love it when this kind of thing happens.

The early years brought lots of joy, lots of challenges but also lots of exhaustion, mentally and physically. I took time off work until Bart was of school age, but even the freedom from that didn't really give enough time in the day to do all that life brought, and there were times when I felt I had given all. A rest, and I would be ready to start again, renewed with the strength to carry on with the job at hand.

When Bart was about three years old, Jane in the physio department stood him against the wall but he couldn't move. 'He will only do it when he is able,' was her reaction and I knew we had to wait! Six months later, I carried Bart to bed and he announced that he wanted to walk! I put him against the bedroom wall, just as Jane had done, and he took his first steps into my arms. What an evening! This was the start of another miracle. I remember him phoning Grandma, saying, 'Grandma, I can walk!' and Grandma cried. I phoned Jane the following morning. The news quickly went around the hospital and there was great excitement in the physio department.

We were absolutely thrilled with this major event, but there was a hard lesson to learn. We had to let go and let him fall. If we hadn't allowed the falls, he would not be walking today. In so many situations in life, we need to let our children go, deal with the bumps and bruises, but enable them to carry on with life's great adventure.

Samuel was a little boy who liked to be close to me and I always wanted to make sure that he had the time and attention he deserved. Regularly people would stop in the street and say, 'How's Bartholomew?' I was always pleased to be asked and for them to show their concern, but tugging at my skirt would be Samuel, just a couple of years older, and I would think, 'If only people would stop and say, "How's Samuel?"' I wanted to make sure that Samuel's experience of the situation was as good as it could be. Time has shown that Samuel has grown up with a tremendous care for the underprivileged and has worked in Africa and shown compassion which has grown partly from his own circumstances. When he was seven, Samuel came home from school with a poem he had written which thrilled us:

My Brother
Brown hair,
Eyes of blue,
Round face,
My brother.

Makes a mess,
Never tidies
Not very strong
My brother.

Likes playing with toys
Always chatting
Fun to be with
My brother

Likes a joke
Always laughing
He's my best friend
My brother

Samuel had piano lessons and the inevitable practising at home gave Bart a strong urge to play. We decided to start with a glockenspiel and I had words with Mrs Carpenter, the piano teacher, about lessons for Bart. I felt that if he learned the music, it could be transferred to piano at a later date if possible. She suggested that I went to the first one and then alternate weeks just to give input on the practical side. The reading came very easily to him and he hammered away with notes for the first two weeks. On the third week he asked, 'Mrs Carpenter, please may I do what you are doing on the piano?' She said she thought, 'What am I going to do? This little boy wants to do what I am doing with both hands and all my fingers accompanying him.' Anyway, she got him on to the piano stool and he was able to press down a note and play with all his might, telling his fingers what to do! My mind went back to when he was born and, trying to look for anything good, I said, 'What lovely long fingers for playing the piano' and the medic attending said, 'He'll never play the piano!' Little by little people will look, and will be amazed!

David's secretary needed a new car and David went to a car auction to bid. We all went but Bart and I decided to sit in the car and what followed was a great moment in Bart's life. Bart asked how he could become a Christian. I explained the gospel to him in very simple language, that God had given His one and only Son for him, and Bart responded. Bart now refers to this time in all of his talks.

There was never any doubt that this was a very real experience for Bart, in spite of the fact that he was only five. Some time later, he was sitting with Grandpa, a devout Christian, and sang to him 'I Want to Serve the Purpose of God (In My Generation)'.

I think everyone in the room battled tears but for Bart it was very genuine, and we see now God's purposes being worked in his life. Because Bart was a Christian, I found some challenging questions easier to deal with. We were on holiday in France when he was still quite young. Samuel and David were scrambling on the rocks and Bart posed the question, 'Am I going to be like this when I'm a man?' My immediate reaction was: 'Bartholomew, I really don't know! What I do know is that the Lord has done all sorts of things for you that weren't supposed to happen and as that is the case, we can expect more things to come.' This was not brushing the question aside, it was saying what I felt in my heart was right. Bart seemed to accept that.

As a family our church was very much the centre of our lives, and growing up both boys were fully involved in what was going on. Bart became a member of Royal Rangers (a kind of Scouts) and he enjoyed the activities very much. The leaders of the group accepted him with open arms and did all they could to provide the extra help he required. I remember one Saturday picking him up from a social evening and found that he had been roller skating! They informed me that they decided not to tell me until afterwards, but he donned a pair of skates just like the others and they held him, one each side, and off they went. I think today Health and Safety might prevent that sort of thing from happening, but he really enjoyed it. Similarly, they helped him on sleepovers and camps and he entered into all the activities with his friends. In taking care of him, they blessed us and him more than they will ever know.

Musical evenings were held at our home as David led the church music. A large number of children played instruments and they were encouraged to join the church music group as soon as they were advanced enough to do so. We had really good times on Saturday evenings followed by the Sunday morning service, and a lot of the children from those days are in touch with Sam and Bart now through social media, many of them still involved in their local churches.

Bart's story is the reason for the book so I will leave him to talk about his own experience and the amazing things that have happened and are happening for him. We wonder at the goodness of God and give glory to Him for the remarkable things that have happened to Bart 'little by little'.

Endnotes

1 See Matthew 7:9-11.

2 A word given that is believed to be from the Lord, see 1 Corinthians 14.

3 Used with permission.

4 Written by Mark Altrogge, Sovereign Grace Music.

Introduction

I was born with arthrogryposis, a rare disability which left me with very restricted mobility. My limbs are severely affected so I have limited movement in both knees with only a 30 degree bend in my left knee, and I am unable to lift my arms much higher than my waist.

This has presented a fair amount of challenges as I've grown up. For example, I am not able to use my hand to lift a drink to my mouth like most other people; can you imagine not being able to do something that simple? Instead I'll often leave my drink on the table and bend down to use a straw, or if it's a cup of tea I can bring my head low to the table and tilt it to my mouth. Not only this, but there are many other things that I have had to develop my own way of doing.

This book is about how God can do anything. The road ahead of me seemed impossible, but with God it was possible.

***

When I was seventeen years old I went to sixth form at Brimsham Green School in Yate, near Bristol. Brimsham Green was a normal secondary school, but they also had a number of disabled children who attended. There were extra staff dedicated to helping these children, and one of them told me that they had received something through the post which I might be interested in about regional trials for disabled athletics, and would I like to have a go? I had never raced against disabled people before and decided it might be quite good fun.

The event was down in Yeovil (approximately 1.5 hours from home) and it took place in three weeks so she said I would need to get my entry form in pretty quickly. I wasn't very fast but I could keep going. So I entered for the 1,500m. I then figured that if I was going all the way to Yeovil, I might as well enter a second race otherwise it will be over too quickly. So I entered the 400m too. You have to bear in mind I had never run 1,500m before. I had walked the distance but never run it, but I was optimistic about it all and thought it would be fine – oh, how naïve I was!

I trained for the event over those three weeks and gradually built up to running 1,500m, which I did twice in practice.

On the day of the event, having arrived in Yeovil, my name was called for the starting line-up of the 1,500m and I had assumed we were going to be put into categories according to our disability. Oh no! There were just three of us. There was me, a guy with cerebral palsy and another who was partially sighted. He could run just like an able-bodied person, he just couldn't see so well where he was going. The phrase This is going to go horribly wrong! ran through my mind.

The race got under way and I was soon way behind the other two. It then occurred to me that the partially sighted man was about to lap me. What if he couldn't see me? Fortunately he ran around me, then the man with cerebral palsy lapped me, then the partially sighted man lapped me again, so I ended up having to run the last lap all on my own.

Coming into the final bend with 200m to go, I hear an announcement over the sound system, 'Could Bart Gee please come to the starting line for the 400m!' I'm thinking, 'I'm on my way!'

Almost as soon as I had finished the 1,500m I had to start the 400m. Do you know what was wrong with the winner of the 400m? He was deaf! My only chance was that he couldn't hear the gun! Not only that, this was his first race and I had already run the best part of a mile. This didn't seem fair. Something else which struck me as rather odd about this event was regarding those competing in wheelchairs. Or rather the fact that they didn't compete in their wheelchairs; there were people who simply got up, ran the 400m – beat me – then sat back down! As you can imagine, that was the only time I took part in that event.

Chapter 1: Putting Your Trust in God

—⁓—

Before going into detail about my story, here are some scriptures which have really helped me over the years.

Matthew 14:22-33 – Jesus walks on the water:

> Immediately Jesus made the disciples get into the boat and go on ahead of him to the other side, while he dismissed the crowd. After he had dismissed them, he went up on a mountainside by himself to pray. Later that night, he was there alone and the boat was already a considerable distance from land, buffeted by the waves because the wind was against it.

> Shortly before dawn Jesus went out to them walking on the lake. When the disciples saw him walking on the lake, they were terrified. 'It's a ghost,' they said, and cried out in fear. But Jesus immediately said to them, 'Take courage! It is I. Don't be afraid.'

'Lord, if it's you,' Peter replied, 'tell me to come to you on the water.'

'Come,' he said.

Then Peter got down out of the boat, walked on the water and came towards Jesus. But when he saw the wind, he was afraid and, beginning to sink, cried out, 'Lord, save me!'

Immediately Jesus reached out his hand and caught him. 'You of little faith,' he said, 'why did you doubt?'

And when they climbed into the boat, the wind died down. Then those who were in the boat worshipped him, saying, 'Truly you are the Son of God.'

I think that when Peter stepped out of the boat and began walking towards Jesus, he must have felt completely out of his comfort zone, and once he began to realise the difficulty of the situation with his own strength and thought to himself that this is impossible, that was when he began to sink and Jesus reached out His hand and caught him.

This shows me that instead of focusing on the difficulty of a situation, we should put our trust in God and ask Him to step in and take control.

I mentioned that Peter must have been out of his comfort zone. I think of this as like being in your own box. You might have everything you need in there. A comfy duvet and pillow, perhaps a TV and games console, a well-stocked fridge, a phone. You feel cosy and content. You know where you are. You don't try to make progress in any way; you are happy with what you have and what you can do. But a box boasts only a small space, and has four walls. A box has limits. God actually challenges us to step outside of our box. He wants us to trust Him. With God it is easier to come out of the box and try new things. He gives us reassurance when we are nervous and unsteady.

God is Omnipotent (All-powerful)

Matthew 19:26:

> Jesus looked at them and said, 'With man this is impossible, but with God all things are possible.'

God is Omniscient (He Knows Everything)

Psalm 147:5:

> Great is our Lord, and abundant in power; his understanding is beyond measure. (ESV UK)

Isaiah 40:28:

> Have you not known? Have you not heard? The LORD is the everlasting God, the Creator of the ends of the earth. He does not faint or grow weary; his understanding is unsearchable. (ESV UK)

God is Omnipresent (He is Everywhere)

Psalm 139:1-18:

> You have searched me, LORD, and you know me. You know when I sit and when I rise; you perceive my thoughts from afar. You discern my going out and my lying down; you are familiar with all my ways. Before a word is on my tongue you, LORD, know it completely. You hem me in behind and before, and you lay your hand upon me. Such knowledge is too wonderful for me, too lofty for me to attain.
>
> Where can I go from your Spirit? Where can I flee from your presence? If I go up to the heavens, you are there; if I make my bed in the depths, you are there. If I rise on the wings of the dawn, if I settle on the far side of the sea, even there your hand will guide me, your right hand will hold me fast. If I say, 'Surely the darkness will hide me and the light become night around me,' even the darkness will not be dark to you; the night will shine like the day, for darkness is as light to you.
>
> For you created my inmost being; you knit me together in my mother's womb. I praise you because I am fearfully and wonderfully made; your works are wonderful, I know that full well. My frame was not hidden from you when I was made in the secret place, when I was woven together in the depths of the earth. Your eyes saw my unformed body; all the days ordained for me were written in your book before one of them came to be. How precious to me are your thoughts, God! How vast is the sum of them! Were I to count them,

they would outnumber the grains of sand – when I awake, I
am still with you.

So if God is omnipotent (all-powerful), omniscient (He knows
everything) and omnipresent (He is everywhere), this shows to
me that God has no limits!

Chapter 2: Age 0 to Four

My disability, arthrogryposis, is a disease of new-borns resulting in decreased flexibility of the joints. Symptoms include weak muscles and stiff joints and this varies drastically from person to person; for example, one person could be affected in their wrist, another in the lower half of their body, or it can affect the whole body. The severity of arthrogryposis differs from person to person and each is uniquely affected.

When I was born, I was severely disabled. The doctors said I would never walk, may never have the strength to be able to sit up independently, and I would have a bleak outlook to life.

I was brought up in a Christian family, and the pastor of our church prophesied to my parents saying, 'Little by little, Bart will be able to do more and more new things that will amaze people.'

He prayed for two things specifically:

1. That one day I would be physically able to walk down the aisle of the church.

2. That one day I would be able to play the organ like my father (my father played the organ most weeks, if not every week, at church and being able-bodied would play with both hands and all of his fingers).

I very much believe that when you ask God to step in, God who is omnipotent, omniscient and omnipresent, so therefore knows no impossibility, He can totally transform a situation that is impossible into something miraculous.

I used to go with Mum to the Bristol children's hospital very regularly for physiotherapy sessions. When I was three years old, I was already able to sit up independently. There was one session in particular where I remember the physiotherapist propped me up against the wall, let go of me and asked me to try to start walking. I couldn't move and I remember feeling frustrated that other children my age were up on their feet and running around and I couldn't move. At that age, I didn't fully understand what my disability meant.

A few months later, Mum was putting me to bed. As she carried me up the stairs, a thought dropped into my head, 'Now you're going to start walking!' It was so clear in my mind, even at that young age. So I said to Mum, 'I think I'm going to start walking now!' So following the example of the physiotherapist, Mum propped me up against the wall. I took three steps and then fell down. We tried again and I took three steps and fell down. I remember feeling very happy. Mum then took me to show my father and brother. Then we phoned my grandparents who were so pleased to hear the news too.

Someone who has a physical disability is often referred to as having physical difficulties. If you take the word 'difficult', what other words have a similar meaning? Maybe 'hard' or 'challenging', for example. Is there a word that sums up 'difficult', 'hard' and 'challenging'? For me, that word is 'possible'!

So for me there was something very significant about the fact that I started by taking three steps; my first step was aided by the wall, then I was able to take two steps independently before I fell down. This meant that both legs were strong enough for me to walk unaided. This was then the start of something 'difficult', 'hard' and 'challenging' – yet it was 'possible'!

The next day it was a matter of seeing if I could get from one side of the room to the other, often getting stuck part way and falling over. Eventually I managed it and I kept on trying to do a little bit more each day until I got to the stage where I could walk in my own way without having to think about it.

Although I had seen many wheelchairs out and about, at the age of three I thought that wheelchairs were for elderly people so I grew up expecting that one day I would walk. Nowadays, thinking that I could have spent my life in a wheelchair makes me truly appreciate that I actually managed to get going on my feet. Life in a wheelchair for me would have been so restricting, bearing in mind the limited mobility I have in my arms too.

Chapter 3: Age Five to Eleven

When I was five, I went to a car auction with my family. Dad and my brother got out and I stayed in the car with Mum. I have no idea what had prompted me to start thinking about God at this moment, but suddenly I realised that I had no doubt, even at that age, about God's existence. So I said to Mum, 'I want to become a Christian. How do I become a Christian?' She firstly told to me the scripture:

> For God so loved the world that he gave his one and only Son, that whoever believes in him shall not perish but have eternal life.
> John 3:16

She then told me that I need to pray and ask Jesus into my heart.

> If you declare with your mouth, 'Jesus is Lord,' and believe in your heart that God raised him from the dead, you will

be saved. For it is with your heart that you believe and are justified, and it is with your mouth that you profess your faith and are saved.
Romans 10:9-10

I have been asked in the past, if God exists, how come He hasn't healed me of my disability?

I do very much believe that God can heal people instantly, but I also believe that God can use people through the difficulty of a situation so that His works can be displayed and for His glory to shine through that person.

Three times I pleaded with the Lord to take it away from me. But he said to me, 'My grace is sufficient for you, for my power is made perfect in weakness.' Therefore I will boast all the more gladly about my weaknesses, so that Christ's power may rest on me. That is why, for Christ's sake, I delight in weaknesses, in insults, in hardships, in persecutions, in difficulties. For when I am weak, then I am strong.
2 Corinthians 12:8-10

***

As I grew up, I was able to take part in many different sports and activities at varying levels of ability including running, football, table tennis and swimming.

When I was eight, I started having swimming lessons at school. In my first lesson, my teacher put a lifejacket on me and came with me into the shallow end of the pool to see if I could swim at all. I had very limited arm movement, but just the very fact that I could move my arms a little bit meant that I could swim very slowly in the water.

At the end of my first lesson, he took my lifejacket off and said, 'I want you to go and swim down to the deep end.' As you can imagine, this was completely out of my comfort zone, but I managed it and I felt such a sense of achievement. I could swim! Sometime after that, he asked me to stand by the side of the pool at the deep end and he wanted me to dive in. He taught me a particular technique as I couldn't lift my arms. I had to fall forwards, head first, and he wanted me to turn while I was under water and come up on my back. I was really fearful about this. I thought, 'What if I can't turn and get stuck upside down?' I would sometimes stand by the side of the pool for twenty minutes trying to have the courage to dive in. One time my instructor actually came along and pushed me in! And actually it wasn't that bad after all. Sometimes I think the thought of diving in was worse than diving in itself. I am so pleased he pushed me outside of my comfort zone as it has opened up so many more opportunities, which I will explore further later on.

Although I couldn't see the outcome of how diving into the pool was going to work, my teacher could, and he had the confidence that I would be able to do it. I think in the same way we can sometimes face a difficult situation and we can't necessarily see the outcome, but we need to ask God to step in, put our trust in Him and let Him take control.

***

I was able to start running when I was five years old and, although I was much slower than an able-bodied person, it meant I was able to take part in various sports. I was always someone who wanted to take part in what I could, rather than watch from the sidelines. At school when we went out to the playing field at break time, I didn't want to watch my friends play football, I wanted to play. My friends were very good at letting me join in; they realised I was slower than them but I loved it, and was glad to be able to take part. Just like anyone else playing football I would occasionally fall down and my friends would come over to help me up and we would carry on playing. Sometimes I would play in goal and other times I would play in an outfield position, often as a defender.

Growing up, I didn't know anyone with the same disability so it meant that if I wanted to take part in sports and activities, I would have to adapt and find my own way. Just because I can't always do things in the same way as an able-bodied person, it doesn't mean I can't do it, I just have to approach the situation and think, 'How can I make this work for me?' Very often there are ways to take part in or accomplish tasks.

Also when I was five years old, we had a piano at home which Dad would play regularly and it really inspired me to want to start learning. As mentioned earlier, the pastor of our church prayed that one day I would be able to play the organ like my dad.

I preferred the sound of the piano to the organ, but it is a similar instrument. When I was very young, we had a meeting with a consultant and Mum asked him, with that little bit of hope, as Dad played the piano and the organ, if there would be any chance of me playing too. The consultant said, looking at my hands as they were, that there was absolutely no chance whatsoever, in fact there was doubt that I would have the strength to even press down a key.

As I really wanted to have a go at playing the piano, my parents agreed for me to try, so they arranged for me to start having lessons to see how I got on. First, my parents and teacher thought it would be worth getting me started on the glockenspiel, an instrument similar to the xylophone, but with a higher-sounding pitch. My teacher would strap the stick to my right hand and then I would try to hold both hands together in order to be able to move the stick around to play different notes. I remember the effort it took me to do this as it meant I would need to lift my hands, something I couldn't do with my hands independently, but with a lot of effort I could do this holding both hands together. In the first few lessons, my teacher taught me some basics in music just to give me a little bit of understanding.

During a lesson as a demonstration, my teacher played a chromatic scale with one hand on the piano. I thought to myself, 'I would love to do that!' So I asked if I could try. My teacher asked me to sit on the piano stool; she pushed the stool in and I was ready to try.

The first thing was, could I press down a key? In my own head I went with the thought that I could do it. I tried with my left hand and I tried with my right hand. So for me, the very fact that

I could press down a key with both hands meant it was the start of something difficult, hard and challenging, and yet it was still going to be possible! I always knew that playing the piano would be a challenge but that is exactly how I wanted to treat it – as a challenge.

In my first few piano lessons, it was a matter of just starting to play using my thumbs. I would play with my right thumb on middle C and my left thumb on C an octave lower.

To start with, it was fairly slow progress but I eventually got to a standard where I could play piano pieces at a very basic level. Although I was taught how to play with standard fingering, I didn't have use of some of my fingers so my teacher would substitute the proper fingering in order to adapt to a way that it would work for me.

When I was eight years old, with my teacher having previously decided that I would not take Grade 1 and 2 piano exams as she was teaching me to play in a very specific way, she decided that I had made enough progress to attempt the Grade 3 piano exam. I passed first time with a Merit.

Around the same time, my teacher decided to enter me for an eisteddfod (a music competition) in Thornbury near Bristol, just a few minutes' drive away from school. There were four of us taking part in the competition. I remember sitting nervously waiting for other musicians to play their pieces. Then it was my turn. I walked over to the piano, put my music in front of me, sat on the stool, and played a piece called 'Alexandra March'. This was my first piano competition and the judge read out the scores. I got 86 per cent, marginally beating the other participants. I won! I was so pleased. This did me the world of good and gave the confidence I needed to progress further.

I was gradually able to do more and more so that by the time I was eleven, I had passed my Grade 5 piano.

I used to attend the Mount of Olives Church in Bristol and I started playing there when I was eight years old as an extra keyboard player as accompaniment to my father and another pianist. As I grew up playing the piano, I always wanted to get to a standard where I could play like an able-bodied pianist and be able to lead worship without my playing being a distraction.

Chapter 4: Age Eleven to Eighteen

Secondary School

I moved to a secondary school near Bristol and the new music teacher was not able to take me on for piano lessons, so having reached Grade 5, I taught myself for a few years. Over these few years, I would work out my own fingering techniques to make the most out of what I could do. I couldn't play with all of my fingers so I needed to develop my own style that would work for me. I felt a real appreciation that I had reasonable movement in my right leg which enabled me to use the sustain pedal while playing.

For both primary and secondary school, my parents felt it would be good for me to go to a normal school where I could be as independent as possible, though I needed some extra help with certain tasks. However, secondary school was quite a challenging time for me, particularly when I was eleven to fifteen years old, as I experienced a lot of bullying. Being disabled, I think I was seen as a weak and easy target and this would encourage people to pick on me. As well as calling me names and spitting at me, children would push me over, knowing that I wasn't able to get up off the floor without help. I found this hard, but I used to try not to let it get me down.

I moved to Brimsham Green School in Yate, near Bristol, for sixth form where I studied Music A-level and GNVQ Information Technology. My experiences of bullying left me incredibly nervous as I walked into the sixth form common room on that first day, feeling vulnerable in front of over 100 strangers. However, my fears were alleviated as some of the students in my form group chose to befriend me. After that, sixth form was a breeze. I really enjoyed my time there and I am still in touch with a few people now, almost twenty years later.

Football

When I was about sixteen years old, I used to go and watch my church football team on Saturday mornings. I thought to myself, 'I would love to be able to take part.' As I had been to watch so many times, I was invited to join in during the warm-up and occasionally I would come on as a substitute. Although I was naturally a defensive player, I would play upfront as a striker due to my lack of speed. It was a great feeling to be able to join in. Twice I had the opportunity to play for ninety minutes.

Chapter 5: Age Nineteen to Present

College

When I was nineteen years old, I applied to go to New Generation Music, a Christian music college in Thornbury near Bristol, only a ten-minute drive from home at the time. I remember going to the audition feeling very nervous. Having listened to me on the piano, they said I could play at a good enough standard to go to the college, but suggested that the course would suit me more if I went to Nexus, another Christian music college, based in Coventry.

I knew that going there would be a big step for me as it would mean I would move away from home for the first time and would need to be relatively independent. But music was my passion and so I applied to enrol on a music and worship course. Amazingly I was accepted straight away.

Moving away from home was becoming a reality and I needed to plan carefully for this. Primarily I needed to arrange a carer.

I knew I was going to attend the Elim Pentecostal Church in Coventry so we contacted the church in advance to see if anyone would be willing to be my carer, and someone accepted.

Having been accepted into the college, it was amazing how everything fell into place. I found out shortly after that there was someone else from my church in Bristol starting the course at the same time. There was someone at my new church in Coventry who I knew from Bristol and when I arrived at the house where I was going to be living, one of my housemates was the brother of one of my old youth leaders. Right from the very start of this new journey God had placed people I knew in each of the three places where I would be spending the most time.

I certainly had my fair share of exercise as I wasn't driving at the time. I lived 0.75 of a mile from the college so just doing this every day meant that I would walk 1.5 miles before doing anything else. This was great for me, though. I loved being active and it gave me time to think and pray about my day.

Studying at Nexus was really where I developed as a musician. A typical day would start with warming up on the piano, and then in our instrument classes we would learn about a particular style of music such as reggae or jazz or classical. We would learn a piece in that style and then follow it up with a Bible study. All the students from the different instrument classes would then meet upstairs in the hall where we would form bands to play the piece of music that we had learned in the morning.

It was great for me to have the opportunity to go to Nexus as it was an opportunity to play with really good musicians and be pushed outside of my comfort zone.

Drumming World Record Attempt

Every year at the college they would do a challenge as part of a fund-raising event. I heard that the drummers were going to do a team endurance drumming world record attempt.

One of the main rules for the attempt was that you had to use three limbs at any one time. I thought, 'I can do that!' Although it's not the standard way to drum, I knew that I could hold a drumstick with two hands and I had good enough use of my right leg to operate the bass drum, so I asked the drummers if I could join them and take part for the world record attempt and they happily let me!

As well as using three limbs all of the time, the other rules were:

- Each song had to be a minimum of two minutes.
- After every song you had a maximum thirty-second break.
- Every eight hours you had a fifteen-minute break.
- At least three people had to be playing at any one time for the record to stand (we couldn't do this in a relay, we either had to keep going or drop out).

Having heard that the current world record was around 27.5 hours, I knew I had good endurance and thought that this was manageable.

We completed a successful eight-hour practice run a few days ahead of the main event, and on the day of the attempt we donned our earplugs and began at 8:30am. There were twelve of us taking part and, as you can imagine, twelve drum kits in a room just big enough to hold us was pretty loud.

The attempt got underway and it was a great feeling to think I was able to take part in it. The local news team came in to film us for a short while during our attempt so that they could broadcast it on the local news.

I realised one of the difficult things for me during the challenge would be eating and drinking. Everyone else could use both feet and one hand to drum and pick up food or drink with their other hand, whereas with my disability I need two hands to pick things up, and if you remember the rules state that we had be using at least three limbs for drumming. So each time we had a thirty-second break at the end of a song, I would quickly put my drumstick down on the snare drum, pick up what I was eating with two hands, take a bite and quickly put it back down so that I could get hold of the drumstick in time for the next song. It took around twenty minutes to eat a chocolate bar!

After the first eight-hour session, I was able to get up and stretch my legs and leave the room for a few minutes before having to go back for the second eight-hour stint. I still had plenty of energy and was ready for the second session. Just like the first session I made it through fairly easily, but I remember walking out of

Bart as a baby

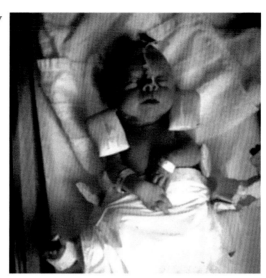

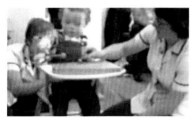

Bart Playing Glockenspiel

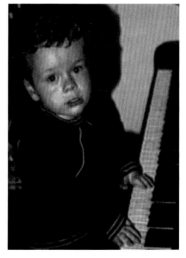

Bart before he could
play the piano

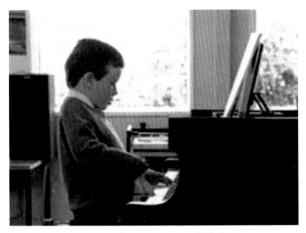

Bart at his piano eisteddfod

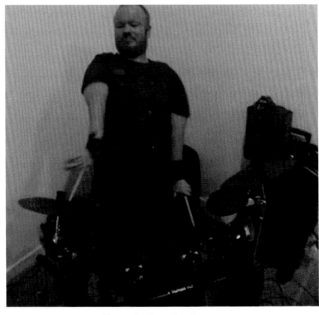

Bart playing the drums

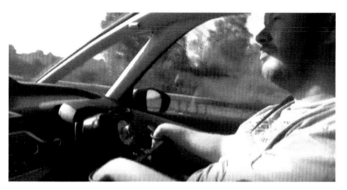

Bart driving his adapted car

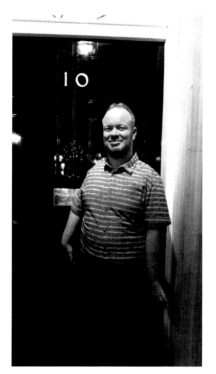

Bart outside No.10 Downing Street

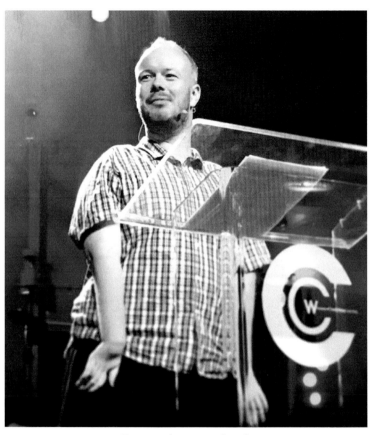

Bart speaking at a church

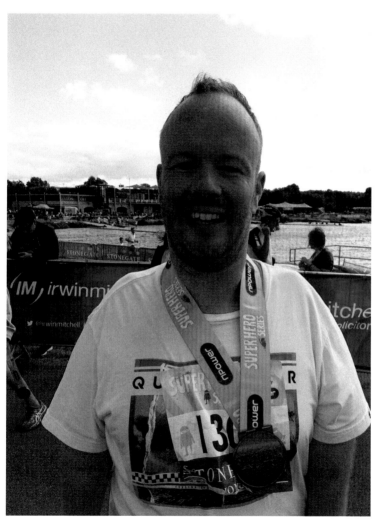

Bart having finished Superhero Triathlon 2017

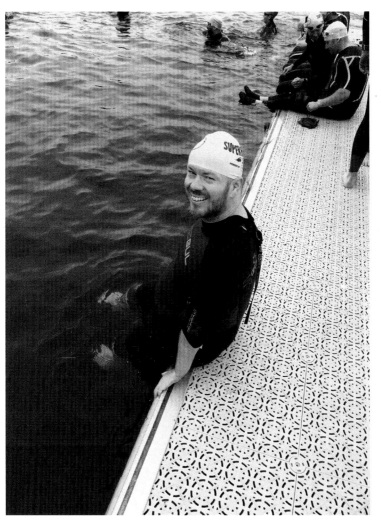

Bart about to start Superhero Triathlon 2018

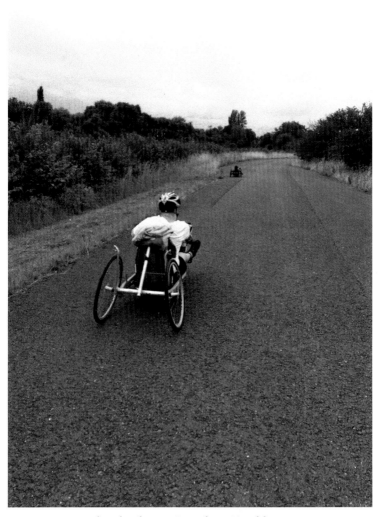
Bart handcycling in Superhero Triathlon 2018

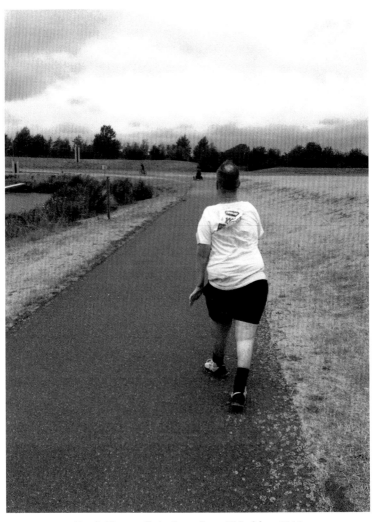

Bart's 5km walk in Superhero Triathlon 2018

the room feeling quite disorientated. The tiredness was starting to set in; that, along with the loud music. The third session was the night session, and now it was just a matter of durability and not falling off my seat in exhaustion. I felt good and allowed the excitement and exhilaration to wash over me.

Having completed three sessions, it was now the following morning. I realised we were not too far away from the world record and I knew from then on that we would make it. So far only two people had dropped out from the twelve that started.

As we approached the world record time of around 27.5 hours, there was a countdown, ten, nine, eight, seven... and we made it! We got the world record! But we weren't going to stop there. We continued to the end of the fourth session. At the fifteen-minute break between the fourth and fifth sessions, we realised that two of the drummers were struggling to keep going. We went for about thirty minutes more and rather than those two having to stop and miss out on beating the world record by six hours we all decided to stop at the same time. Our final time was thirty-three hours and thirty-three minutes.

On the one hand I was thrilled to have got the world record but I'll admit I was a little disappointed that we stopped when we did as I was feeling quite good and had a lot left in the tank.

Unfortunately, three weeks after we got the record, another group smashed our record. Go figure. But at least I can say I was a world record holder for three weeks, and I would be ready to do it again!

Playing Drums and Bass Guitar

I had always liked the bass guitar as an instrument and it suddenly occurred to me, at the age of eighteen, how I could play it. I knew that I wouldn't be able to hold it with the strap on as I wouldn't have the strength in my fingers to press down the strings. So I came up with an idea. I realised that I would be able to put the bass guitar flat on a keyboard stand – a similar position to someone playing the Hawaiian guitar – and as long as I was standing up I could get enough downward pressure on the strings with my left hand to change the notes and pluck with my right hand. I had developed an ear for music and it came quite naturally to me what notes I should play. I could only play at a fairly basic level, but this was at least another instrument I could play. I think it would be easy for others as well as myself to simply assume that playing the bass guitar was just something that I wasn't able to do, but it just goes to show that some limitations are only in our heads. Even if something is difficult, it is still possible.

I wasn't yet content with my technique for playing the drums. I had previously played holding a stick with two hands so that I could play just using the bass and snare drum. But I felt I could do better and wanted to find a way to play the drums properly. At the gym I would wear wristbands – a bit like you see with tennis players. It occurred to me that I could wear two on each arm and tuck the sticks inside to help hold them in place. To compensate for the limited movement in my arms, I would sit high up on a stool which gave me the mobility I needed to be able to play.

Just like with the bass guitar, I taught myself and for the first couple of weeks I could use both of my hands for the hi-hat and snare drum. However, as soon as I tried to add the bass drum by using my right foot, I would struggle with the coordination. With practise I gradually got used to it and could soon play a basic but authentic drum rhythm. Once I was able to play some different drum patterns, I started playing along to music; not very well at first, but I gradually improved and was eventually able to keep time and do drum fills.

Some Limits Are OK

Unfortunately, having finished the year at Nexus, I needed to return home as I had developed arthritis in my ankles. It became quite severe and I needed to have ankle surgery to stop the pain. It took a long time to recover from both ankle operations and it was around eighteen months before I was able to walk long distances again. The surgery really helped but it meant that I had to give up running, football and anything that put a lot of pressure on my ankles. I was pretty frustrated about this because I had always worked so hard to break the boundaries and limitations of my physical circumstances. This felt like going backwards. It felt like I had failed somehow. Doctors had said I would be lucky to walk, to have any quality of life, and I had proved them so wrong. But now arthritis had come into play and was trying to stop me from doing the things I loved to do. I came to realise that actually it's OK if I can't do everything. I believe God can do anything, and that He can smash all obstacles in front of me. But maybe there's a reason He's not smashing them all right now. Sometimes we have to be patient and wait for Him. Sometimes He wants us to focus on something else for now. I learned to concentrate on other things that bring me joy.

I moved on by swimming regularly. This was low impact and good for my joints and at least it kept me active. I didn't want to give up sport altogether, but I wanted to find things to do where it wouldn't be a problem for my ankles. I started going to the gym to keep me fit during recovery and I would focus on working the upper body. Then someone suggested I should try cycling; however, I didn't have enough mobility in my knees to rotate the pedals, but it did give me the idea to look into getting a handcycle. I went to a shop to try it out and I realised it was going to work if I could adapt it. I always knew I would be slower than an able-bodied person on a bike, but I could still go for rides as long as it was relatively flat.

I would quite often go on bike rides with friends, often on the Bristol to Bath cycle track. One of my first rides was with a friend who had a dog, a husky. To help me go faster, my friend attached the dog to the front of my bike using a rope. What could go wrong, right? Of course, as is often the nature of our beloved canine friends, he would want to chase things. In this case it was an unsuspecting squirrel. Brakes on!

New Orleans Trip

In the summer of 1999, when I was seventeen, I went on holiday with my parents to the USA. Having been a number of times previously, we decided to go to the south, to Louisiana and Texas. For our first week, we stayed in Mandeville, Louisiana, on the north side of Lake Pontchartrain, across the water from New Orleans.

Having arrived on the Saturday, we searched for a church and came across Victory Fellowship, a church of around 2,000 people in New Orleans. We decided to go there in the evening, and when we arrived I was invited to go to the youth service in the building next door. As soon as I walked in I felt very welcome and quickly made friends and chatted with some of the youth leaders. As it happened, they were holding a week of worship services for the youth. They invited me along for the full week and by the end it, it felt like we were all old friends.

All of this demonstrates that even though I am different because of my disability, I can still fit in and be offered some amazing opportunities. The youth leaders asked me if I would like to come to stay with them during the following summer. I was able to go fishing in the Gulf of Mexico and go on a swamp tour with the other church youth. At least fifty alligators laid before me, their eyes reflecting in the moonlight at 2am. Experiences like this show me that being 'normal' isn't the most important thing. I don't need to be like everyone else to have a full life.

The following summer I went back again, this time for two weeks, and we went tubing. This involves climbing into a rubbing ring tied to the back of a boat and being dragged along behind it. Great fun. And it's the driver's job to try to throw participants out of the ring. Most people ended up in the water. Then it was my turn! As you can imagine, with my limited mobility, I had a little bit of difficulty getting from the boat into the ring. With a lot of help, I managed to get in... only I wound up facing backwards. Never mind. The driver asked me to raise my hand if I need to stop. I said that I couldn't lift my hand but I could kick my right foot, and this was accepted as a reasonable substitute. I asked him not to go too fast to start with as I wasn't sure if I could hold on. He gradually accelerated and we got faster and faster until we were going about 25mph. At this point I realised it would hurt if I fell off, so I resolved to stay on. Then the driver started zigzagging, which further increased my speed and the ring began jumping across the wake of the boat.

Fortunately, because I rely on the rest of my body normally where I can't necessarily use my limbs to do certain tasks, my core upper body is very strong and I was able to shift my body position accordingly to try to keep the rubber ring stable. We got to one end of the lake and the boat slowed down. I was feeling rather pleased with myself for managing to stay on for so long, but as I was facing the wrong direction, I did not realise the driver was doing a U-turn in order to continue the ride! A sudden burst of acceleration took me by surprise, but I managed to keep the ring stable and stayed on for the whole time, around ten minutes in total. I was one of only two people who managed to stay on the ring the whole time; the other four fell in. The reality was that my disability actually made me more capable of certain things than my able-bodied friends. I was a superior competitor in this activity because I had practised using my core so much as a daily part of life.

Although being born able-bodied, or 'normal', would have been great, I can see that my disability can actually contribute positively to my life. The physical disadvantages are many, and they are frustrating, but at the same time I have discovered numerous ways to overcome them, and even found ways that I am physically better than an able-bodied person. But that's just from a physical perspective. In order to overcome the drawbacks of my disability, I have had to develop a lot of resilience (mental strength), I have had to be resourceful, proactive, inventive and brave. So in many ways my disability has shaped my personality to incorporate a lot of positive qualities.

On the final day I was asked to share my story at the evening youth service. I was pretty terrified of speaking in front people at the time, but I felt touched that they wanted to know more about me. Nineteen-year-old me inarticulately blundered through my life story, trying to keep it all relevant and interesting. Their response was understated but encouraging. They understood that I was not comfortable in the spotlight, but they showed me that they valued me and appreciated my testimony.

Driving

When I was twenty-four years old, I wanted to start learning to drive. Because of the limited movement in my limbs and poor grip with my hands, it meant that I would need to have a car adapted, so I went to Motability, a scheme for disabled people.

After an initial assessment, we decided to spread the controls so that I would operate the car using my head, hands and right foot. I knew I would need an automatic car but fortunately I have enough movement in my right leg to operate the accelerator and brake. I have handlebars just like riding a bike with loops so that I can slot my wrists inside and have a proper grip. I also have a button on my headrest which operates the horn, indicators, windscreen wipers and lights on a bleeper system, so you hold the button down for the number of bleeps you want; for example, one bleep for the horn, two bleeps for left indicator, three bleeps for the right indicator, and so on up to ten bleeps. This worked really well for me.

So once I had the vehicle adapted, which took some time, I started having driving lessons. There was a driving instructor at my church who taught people with disabilities and so I had a two-hour lesson with him once a week and Dad would also take me out to get practice.

During one lesson in Weston-super-Mare I was driving down a one-way road and three police motorbikes overtook me. As I was approaching a roundabout my driving instructor asked me to turn right, which meant I needed to change lanes. As soon as he had given the instruction, the last of the police bikes stopped in the second lane and was waving the traffic through. I hesitated and asked my instructor if I should still take the second exit or take the first exit to get out of the way, at which point the policeman shouted at me for taking too long as there was a police convoy catching up with me – they were escorting the Queen! I got told off for holding up the Queen. Oops!

Learning to drive offered me such freedom. I passed my test with two minors, though I do make the occasional mistake, such as pressing the control on my headrest only once instead of twice to indicate and blasting my horn at a police van. Unfortunately, in October 2010 I developed epilepsy which meant that I had to surrender my driving licence. I began having seizures on occasions and wasn't able to drive for two years. Once my epilepsy was being well-managed I was able to get my licence back, but unfortunately there were some blips which meant I had to give up driving for another two years. This was like the arthritis all over again. I was devastated. I had been independent, self-reliant, I'd had freedom. And another illness came along and took it from me! I found this quite frustrating. I didn't even care about the epilepsy itself, I just cared about driving.

In April 2015, I finally got my car and I haven't looked back since. I love driving and I go all over the country when I speak at churches and schools. It gives me a great amount of joy to have that independence back.

Challenges

As you've probably gathered already, I like challenges. And in 2014 I got involved in a local swimathon for Sport Relief. I could do the 1.5km, 2.5km or 5km. I could already swim a mile, so I set myself the challenge of doing the 2.5km swim, which equates to 100 lengths of a normal public swimming pool. I trained for this over a few weeks and wanted to make sure I could swim at least 2km in the build-up to the challenge. I then managed to complete the 2.5km Sport Relief Swimathon in around two hours five minutes.

Having completed that challenge, I wanted to push myself even further and take the next step up, the 5km swimathon. I knew that this would be a real challenge for me physically and mentally. If you think that a length (25m) takes me over a minute, it can get quite boring in a swimming pool trying to complete 200 lengths. So in 2016, I trained really hard for the 5km swim and I would try to swim twice a week. I was limited to time restrictions at whichever leisure centre I used, but on Monday nights the Activity Zone Leisure Centre in Malmesbury, Wiltshire was available for four hours in the evening which meant I had the opportunity to increase my fitness and test my endurance. I gradually built up and my aim the week before the actual swim was to complete 3.8km, the equivalent distance for the swim on an ironman triathlon. This took a couple of months of training but I made it. A week before the event, I had a phone call from Sport Relief. They had received my entry form for the event and had seen that I am physically disabled. They asked a little bit about me, and then asked me what I was doing the following Tuesday. I was invited to No 10 Downing Street for a Sport Relief function as a member of the public who was taking on the challenge. It was such a surprise and, of course, I said I would very much like to go.

They asked me how I would get there, if I would be using public transport or drive. I said I would find it easier to drive and park close by. They then offered to book me a parking space and I was thinking this would be in a car park close to Downing Street.

The next day, I received an email from them saying they had booked me a parking space in Downing Street behind the houses. I couldn't believe it! I was asked if I could bring my passport with me as photo identification.

So on the Tuesday, I drove to London and arrived outside the gates of Downing Street. Groups of tourists with cameras were waiting outside the gates ready to take photos of people driving in and out of Downing Street and there I was about to drive in.

Having checked my passport ID, the police opened the gates and I drove in up to a barrier where they had to do a security check. I put my window down and asked a policeman where I needed to go to park my car. He went off to check and came back and told me to park down the end by the Jaguar. So I drove along Downing Street with No 10 on my right and the cameras on my left and parked next to the Jaguar – David Cameron's Jag, I hasten to add! I got out of the car and walked into No 10. I was taken up to the function room and I realised when I got there that I was one of four members of the public invited, there was also a school class and a number of celebrities involved with Sport Relief including Marvin (formerly part of JLS) and Rochelle Humes (The Saturdays) and Ore Oduba (BBC Sports presenter) who later that year won BBC's Strictly Come Dancing, around fifty of us in total. It seemed such a privilege to get invited.

Mr Cameron soon made an appearance. He circulated among us and asked me about my challenge, and even asked me to stand next him for the group photo. Win!

As part of my swimming training was at the Cotswold Leisure centre in Cirencester, Gloucestershire, I got to know the staff and they were particularly interested in how I was able to swim. Having got to know the staff, I showed my interest in attempting the 5km swimathon. The time limit for the event was three hours but I knew that there was no way I would complete it within the time allowed. The staff were really helpful, they really wanted me to attempt it too and they set up a lane specially for me in the afternoon so that I could be well into my swim before everyone else started.

I had never swum 5km before so it was a bit of an unknown to me. I had no problems in the first half of the swim and it was going really well. But once I had completed 3km I was starting to feel unwell and the further I went, the worse I felt. I was eventually told that I needed to pull out. I was frustrated because I was so close to finishing it (I had completed 182 lengths – 4.55km) but I knew I had to accept their decision. This was a huge disappointment for me, but I knew I would try again. We all face failure. We all get frustrated. I had smashed the world record for drumming, I had passed my driving test, I could play the keyboard and drums, and the bass. I just needed more training!

More importantly, it is so important that we do not equate our value with our accomplishments. Our worth is found in God, who made us. There is nothing we can do to make God love us any more or any less than He already does.

The Bible says, 'Are not five sparrows sold for two pennies? Yet not one of them is forgotten by God. Indeed, the very hairs of your head are all numbered. Don't be afraid; you are worth more than many sparrows' (Luke 12:6-7).

Sparrows used to be sold at the market for little; they were not considered to have much value by people. But Jesus is illustrating here that God still cares for them. His love is unconditional. It does not matter what we can or can't do physically, it does not matter what we look like. He loves us anyway.

Swimathon 2017

Even though I didn't manage to complete the 5km swimathon in 2016, I didn't want to give up on it and so in 2017 I attempted it again. This time it was for Marie Curie cancer.

This time I completed it. Because of my disability, I have very restricted movement in my limbs so I knew it was going to take a long time and I finished it in around five hours thirty minutes. Just the very fact that I have some movement in my limbs enabling me to swim slowly meant that although it was going to be a massive challenge for me, it was still going to be possible, and that's how I try to approach all of my challenges.

I have also completed a number of open water swims which I love doing. I find it so much more enjoyable than just swimming lengths of a pool, as you feel like you are actually going somewhere while swimming. My first attempt at an open water swim didn't go too well. It was 14C in the water and quite choppy. It suddenly occurred to me with it being quite rough in the water that it was a bit more daunting and less safe than the comfort of being in a pool. I had to pull out of the swim not feeling well.

A couple of years later I decided to give it another try and this time it was calm in the water and I absolutely loved it, and have done a number since. If it wasn't for my swimming teacher pushing me outside of my comfort zone when I was young, I may not have had the courage to go open water swimming.

Just because you fail at something the first time, should you give up or try again? Sometimes I don't manage a task the first time but my mindset is that if there is something I really want to do, I won't give up, I will keep trying and trying.

Wiltshire Big Pledge Challenge

Having seen on Twitter that I was a keen swimmer, one of the organisers of the Wiltshire Big Pledge Challenge contacted me about taking part in the summer of 2016. It's an eight-week challenge and there were a number of different options to choose from. As I am able to do as much swimming as I like, I entered the 50km in eight weeks challenge. I knew this was going to be tough for me as I need carers to take me swimming so that I can have help with getting changed. I was only able to go twice a week. Knowing that I would be on holiday for some of the challenge, I was able to swim every day so I made the most of it and most days I swam a mile (1.6km). I managed to finish the challenge with three days to spare.

Having completed the 50km in eight weeks challenge, one of the organisers asked me if I would like to be one of the 'champions' to help promote the Big Pledge Challenge for the summer of 2017. I said that I would very much like to be a part of it and I was asked if I could attend the media launch where I met Great Britain Paralympic swimmer, Stephanie Millward, MBE, who is also based in Wiltshire. While I was at the media launch, I was asked if I could give a five-minute live interview for BBC Radio Wiltshire to try to inspire others to take part.

Having taken part in the media launch, I signed up for the challenge and again needed to choose something that would suit me. I had already entered my first triathlon in August 2017 so I decided to enter the sports challenge which meant that I had to complete 750km in eight weeks, a combination of handcycling, walking and swimming, the three disciplines of the triathlon. I was able to include handcycling in the gym as part of this. I calculated beforehand what I would need to do per day to complete it and I managed to finish the 750km challenge on the final day.

Superhero Triathlon

On 19 August 2017, I attempted the Superhero Triathlon, the first triathlon in the UK specially organised for disabled people of varying disabilities to take part. There were three distances to choose from and you could either do it on your own or as part of a team. I wanted to attempt the longest distance they offered, the equivalent of a sprint triathlon for able-bodied people – 750m swim, 20km handcycle and 5km walk. I knew that this would be a big challenge for me, but I knew that I could do the distances individually so it was a matter of combining the three disciplines. The Wiltshire Big Pledge Sports Challenge was very good training for this triathlon and meant I was fit to attempt it.

Just like the athletics story, I had the worst mobility out of everyone who attempted the longest distance but I managed to complete it in just over four hours (4:12:47). The next slowest person beat me by about one hour thirty minutes. For me, it wasn't about the fact of coming last, it was just brilliant that there was an event like this that I was able to take part in. I attempted the same triathlon again in August 2018 and I just beat my time by sixteen seconds. It was so close! I have entered the race again in August 2019 and I will aim to beat my time, even if it still means I finish last.

As I am always looking for more challenges, I would love at some point to attempt the Olympic distance triathlon though this would take me a very long time (1,500m swim, 40km handcycle and 10km walk).

Tall Ship

When I was around twenty-four years old, I had the opportunity to go on a tall ship for a week. This was with the Jubilee Sailing Trust who had two tall ships at the time specially designed for disabled people to go on.

Another disabled person from my church had previously been away for a week with the Jubilee Sailing Trust and he really enjoyed it and got a lot out of it. So when I was given the opportunity to go, I jumped at it. Each disabled person had to take a carer with them and one of my friends was used to caring at the time so he came with me. We went on the Lord Nelson and our week was in the Canary Islands.

It was a four-hour flight from Bristol to Gran Canaria and someone from the Jubilee Sailing Trust came to meet us at the airport when we arrived. We were then taken about twenty minutes' drive from the airport to the coast where we met the rest of the team and got onto the tall ship. Although the mast was high (approximately 100ft) I was quite surprised how small the ship was. There were two levels on board, the main deck and the bedrooms below with a main room where we would have our meals and any briefings and meetings.

I soon realised that we would have to do shift work. We were split into a number of teams and each team was designated certain hours to be on watch overnight, whether we were out at sea or in port.

For the first night, we stayed in port and then the next morning we went out to sea, gradually to work our way to Santa Cruz in Tenerife. Being the Atlantic Ocean, the sea was quite choppy and on our tall ship we were bobbing up and down. Some of us who were not used to sailing were certainly feeling it, including myself, and it wasn't long until all I could do was lie down on my bed. I did not feel well. Eventually I got used to the movement and within two days we made it to Santa Cruz.

One thing my friend had told me who had previously been on a sailing trip was his experience of climbing the mast. Everyone who wanted to climb it had the opportunity to try. This was something I was really looking forward to doing. Heights did not bother me as long as I knew I was secure. So a number of people went up one-by-one and then it was my turn. For me, I knew it was going to take a lot of physical effort. I had help to put a harness on and two people offered to come up the mast with me, one on each side. The rest of my team were then holding onto the rope at the bottom so that each time I went to push to get up the next step, they would pull on the rope to help me up. Some of the steps were knee-height, which made it very difficult for me with my limited knee movement. It meant that I would have to let go of the ladder with my hands, completely relying on the harness by leaning to the left just so that I could try to get my right foot up onto the next step. It was such an effort. It took me about forty-five minutes to climb 30ft of the mast. I was shattered but I had made it that far. It was such a great feeling being that high up and actually making it up that high, even though I needed the help. Before climbing the mast I had eaten a cooked breakfast. By the time I was back down again I felt like I could eat another, I had used up such a lot of energy.

Throughout the week, we would be working all day and some of the time we would be out on watch during the night so it was a matter of grabbing some sleep when I could.

Breaking Limits

In 2014, I was invited to share my story at Bristol Brunel Academy, a secondary school in Bristol. I arrived at the school not knowing if I would be going into classrooms or assemblies. At the time, I used to find speaking in front of people quite nerve-racking and it was something I wouldn't normally do, but as I was invited into the school, I agreed to it. I remember arriving at the school feeling very nervous.

I arrived at the school finding out that I was taking three assemblies, first for Year 9, then Year 8 and finally Year 7, a total of around 650 children. I was asked if I could share my story and play the piano for them.

After each assembly I had children coming up to ask me questions and they stood around me wanting to watch how I played the piano. I heard later that there were some students wanting to start learning the piano having watched me play.

There were two things that really stood out to me that day:

First, there was a boy from Year 8 who came up to me and all he said quietly was, 'Sir, I think you're amazing.' It wasn't until later that evening I had a message from the teacher who invited me in saying she could not believe the boy said that to me as he was the worst behaved boy in the year and was on report to her.

Secondly, there was a girl who came up to me after the Year 7 assembly saying that as soon as I started playing the piano, she started to cry. This was because her mother had some sort of disability and had basically given up trying to cope with it. She said after seeing me, she was going to go home and talk to her mother about me and was going to try to motivate her after what I said.

Just these two things made me start to think, 'Although I find it hard talking in front of people, with the impact it made at Bristol Brunel Academy, is this something I should be doing on a more regular basis?'

It took me a while but in November 2015, I was invited to share my story at Bethel Church in Oldbury, Birmingham. I had great feedback and received this testimonial from the Reverend Helen Robertson, the pastor of the church:

> If you have ever wrestled with your 'Why God?' moments, then Bart's journey of grace is something you need to hear! Life's struggles get put back into perspective when Bart

tells his story and you realise again that nothing, absolutely nothing is impossible with God!

In December 2015, I was invited into another school and again had a really good response from the children, and I really felt this was something that I should start doing regularly.

So I decided to create a website www.breakinglimits.co.uk with the title 'Breaking Limits' and 'Turning Disability Into Possibility' as the slogan. My reason for calling it 'Breaking Limits' is that doctors said I would never walk, may never sit up independently and would have a bleak outlook to life, but when you ask God to step in, God who knows no impossibility, I believe He can totally transform a situation that is impossible in our eyes into something possible, therefore limits are broken and miracles happen.

As I wasn't known to a lot of people, it took a while for the ministry to get going and I did only six talks in the first six months, but I have gradually seen opportunities open up and I am now speaking very regularly around the UK in churches, schools and other organisations.

I had quite an experience in March 2017. I was invited to speak at Vinney Green Secure Unit for young offenders in Bristol. I had a briefing beforehand and was told that just because I was disabled, it wouldn't necessarily mean they wouldn't be abusive towards me. I was asked if I could speak to groups of four and plan to do forty-five-minute sessions with them, the same session four times with different groups. I was told that some of the offenders had committed some of the most serious crimes so I realised that this was going to be a challenge.

When I arrived, I spoke with the headteacher before the day started and he said to me that although I had planned to do forty-five-minute sessions, I shouldn't expect it to last more than five or ten minutes as the offenders would stop it when they wanted it to end.

The offenders were not made to sit down and I remember in my first session, there was a boy around fourteen years old and as I was talking he would slowly walk around the room, not looking like he was interested, and gazing out of the window. Without warning, as I was speaking he came and walked close beside me, then stood behind me. He was trying to intimidate me and wanted to see if I trusted him. I didn't react, knowing that there were other staff in the room who could intervene if necessary.

I broke the forty-five-minute session into different sections, hoping to keep their attention. I spoke for ten minutes, then showed a video which demonstrated how I had adapted to take part in various activities.

At that point, the boy who tried to intimidate me sat down to watch the video and then watched me play the keyboard. After that, I got the offenders that wanted to, to do a task as if they have my disability. I would get them to sit down on the floor and ask them to get up without bending their legs or using their hands. None of them could do it. So I asked them to imagine if they had fallen over in the room and there was no-one around to help them up, they didn't have a phone, and they couldn't call for help, what were they going to do?

One said they would lie down and go to sleep!

I showed them how I would get up. There were a number of seats in the room so I shuffled over to one by a wall so that the seat wouldn't move. I would lean against the chair using my legs to support me but having to rely on my back and stomach muscles. Once I had managed to get up onto the seat, I realised the seat was too low for me to stand up. I would then have to lean against the wall using my legs to support me and push up with my back and stomach muscles. I managed it and the offenders saw how difficult it was. I then asked the offenders if they would like to give it a go and most of them tried it. They all found it hard but it gave them an understanding of when something is 'difficult', 'hard' or 'challenging', it is still 'possible'.

I then did a question and answer session and I was asked a number of questions. This showed me that they were focused and actually getting something out of the session. If they were not interested at all, they would not have asked questions, so for me it was great that they were actually responding to me. At the end of the session we set up table tennis and pool tables and, having watched me play table tennis on the video, one of the offenders immediately asked me to have a game with him. I explained to him that as I have poor grip, I have to hold the bat with two hands and can therefore only manage backhand shots. Some rallies he won and some I won. I then played pool with the boy who had previously tried to intimidate me. He was very polite towards me. He would say, 'Good shot!', 'Thanks' and 'Cheers' when I passed the cue back to him, as we had to share it. It was great to see the change in him between the start and end of the session.

At lunch time, all the staff would sit with the offenders; there needed to be two sittings as some offenders were not able to be in the same room as other offenders at the same time.

Having finished my food, one offender who had previously been in one of my sessions offered to get me a dessert. After lunch, another offender saw I was having difficulty getting up from my chair and he immediately came over to help me. Staff were really surprised at this and it shows how well they responded to me.

At the end of one of the sessions, one of the offenders went out of the room almost in tears.

I ended up taking four forty-five minute sessions without any problems whatsoever.

I imagine they responded so well to me because they could relate to me. In their own lives, they have their problems and to them it may seem like they are facing a brick wall. They watched me come in and saw how I faced my problems or difficulties and could see how I took them on and didn't give in.

If by going into the young offenders' unit it had an impact on one person, it would certainly be worth it!

I was invited back to speak Vinney Green Secure Unit again in February 2018. Nearly all of the offenders were new, only two had been in my session from last year. This time I had to take six forty-five minute sessions, the same session as the previous year in the same format. It was very interesting when I came to the task where they had to get up off the floor as if they have my disability because in one of the sessions, two of the offenders remembered the challenge from the year before. One offender who knew how I managed the task helped the other offenders by encouraging them to think how to approach the challenge. This was great for me to see how he responded because the staff at the unit said it was very difficult to get him to respond.

The head of Vinney Green Secure Unit has said he would like me to go again once he has another group of people I can speak to.

Funny Train Story

Because of the difficulty I have with walking and the stiffness and weakness in my legs, it means that I have poor balance. This can occasionally get me into some embarrassing, awkward or funny situations.

I would have been aged thirty-three or thirty-four years old and I remember getting onto a train at Bristol Temple Meads station to go home from work. I entered the carriage and walked down the aisle to find an available seat. As I walked past the table seats, I lost my balance. Of course, with my disability I am not able to put my hands out in front of me to stop myself. To her surprise, I fell across a woman's lap and I ended up lying horizontally, wedged between her and the table as she was trying to eat a sandwich. I was so embarrassed! You should have seen the look on her face. She was shocked! The next thing I thought was, 'I can't get up!' All I could think of to do was to move down onto the floor of the aisle and I shuffled along to an available seat where I could get myself up. Fortunately, she was absolutely fine about it, to my relief.

Relationships

One thing I have struggled with over many years is, why would someone marry me as a disabled person when they could be with an able-bodied person? I know I shouldn't think like this but I have found this quite hard. I think having a disability is a barrier for a lot of people, but I hope one day that someone will love me for who I am and I will one day get married. I believe that God's timing is perfect and I have to put my trust in Him.

Living with My Disability

As you can see from some of my stories, I like to live an active lifestyle and I try not to let my disability get in the way and want to take part in as much as possible. For me, it is not so much of a problem that I am slower than able-bodied people at taking part in sports and activities, but I see it more as a challenge to improve so that I can keep up, or at least not be too far behind everyone else.

I am very happy as a person. I have lived with my disability all of my life, with all the difficulties and challenges, but this for me is normal. I know I look different to an able-bodied person but I feel normal – it is just my 'normal' is a bit different from everyone else's 'normal'.

Although it would be very interesting to know what it is like to be able-bodied, it does not matter at all to me that I am disabled. It is part of who I am.

Music and Worship: Breaking Your Limits – the Pieces of the Puzzle

In any challenge I attempt, I don't go in with a 'can't do!' attitude. If there is something I really want to do, I think to myself, 'What if I could?' If something looks really difficult to be able to achieve, is there a way around the difficulty, and how can I improve? Remember, when something is difficult, hard or challenging, with God it is still possible!

Music and worship is a big part of my life. When my parents were told by the doctor that there would be no chance whatsoever that I would be able to play the piano or the organ and even doubt that I would have the strength to press down a key, just the very fact that I could press down a key with both hands meant it was possible, so I really saw playing the piano as a challenge.

Having passed my Grade 5 aged eleven, I really wanted to get to a standard where I could play the piano in church without my playing being a distraction to the congregation and other band members. I realise that God 'looks at the heart' (1 Samuel 16:7) but I also want to be able to play to the best of my ability, and I always look for ways to improve.

These two scriptures are the reason I want to play to the best of my ability and to continue to develop as a musician.

Psalm 103:1:

> Bless the LORD, O my soul, and all that is within me, bless his holy name! (ESV UK)

Psalm 33:3:

> Sing to him a new song; play skilfully, and shout for joy.

Although worship is not just music, music is a way we can express our worship to God. In the world, we may all speak different languages, but no matter which country you are from, you can always express your worship to God through music.

My reason for wanting to improve as a musician all the time is so that I can play 'all that is within me' in my worship to God.

Maybe you have got to a point where you can play your instrument to a standard but you don't know how to improve further. Think about this – music is endless, it doesn't matter if you are the best musician in the world, there are still ways you can improve, no matter your ability.

Two words that jump out at me from Psalm 33:3 are 'play skilfully'. So how can you improve or develop as a musician?

This is a concept that I use. Try to think of music like a jigsaw puzzle. If I was doing a jigsaw puzzle, I wouldn't approach it piece by piece but I would separate the pieces into sections, for example, one section would be the edge pieces, another section would be the buildings, another, the sky, and another, a river. By separating the pieces into sections before even attempting the puzzle means that I can focus on one section at a time.

So how do you relate music to a jigsaw puzzle?

I would break up music into different sections:

Primary example – music

- learning musical scales (major and minor)
- melody
- harmony
- aural – playing by ear
- rhythm

Secondary example – or, if your challenge is related to exercise, your sections of the puzzle might look like this:

- endurance
- strength building
- speed etc.

You may have fewer or more sections in your challenge.

Each of these sections could be seen as different parts of the puzzle, for example, learning musical scales could be the edge pieces, the melody could be the buildings, harmony could be the sky, etc.

So let's take each of the above musical sections to demonstrate how you could improve your musical ability if progressing your skills is part of your challenge.

Don't get overwhelmed by the big picture, but focus on the shorter-term goals and seeing the big picture as motivation only.

Learning Musical Scales

Think of each musical scale as a language, for example C Major could be English, D Major could be French, E Major, Spanish, and so on.

Many of you who play the piano probably would have started playing in C Major as there are no sharps or flats, just the white keys on the piano. But say you want to transpose what you are playing from C Major to G Major. You may use a number chart to do this. I think of a number chart like a dictionary. A number chart is used to transpose from one key to another just like a dictionary is used to translate from one language to another.

However, just like learning a new language, the more you practise a musical scale in a particular key, the more fluent you become, which means that you are able to start thinking in the new key you are playing in rather than having to rely on the number chart. Think of each musical scale as an edge piece; for each musical scale you can play it is another edge piece joined together. Once you are able to play every scale fluently, all the edge pieces are joined together.

Likewise, if your goal is sport-related, this section could be about improving your endurance. Each puzzle piece could be the different exercises you do to improve in different ways (e.g. squat longer than run). Also practise.

Melody

Once you have learned all of the major and minor scales, try taking a song you know well in the key of C Major. Take the melody, preferably a simple melody to start, and see if you can play it in the key of G Major, then the key of D Major and so on until you are able to play this melody in any key. This may seem difficult to start with, but the more you practise the melody in each key, the easier it will become and you will gradually see progress, therefore you are now starting to join together the buildings' pieces.

Harmony

Now that you can transpose a melody into any key, you can start working on the harmony. Take a simple song which has four or five chords in total. First, play the song in C Major, then having learned your scales, see if you can transpose the chords to G Major, then D Major and so on until you can play these chords in any key. Each time you can play the chords in a new key, you are joining two sky pieces together. Can you see the progress you are making?

No matter how good a musician you are, you can always do things to improve. If you are an accomplished musician and this is easy for you, try taking a song and see if you can use alternative chords to support the melody. Experiment with jazz chords; this is something I like to do in my own time. The more you do, the more sky pieces you are joining together.

Aural – playing by ear

Knowing your musical scales is really helpful for being able to play by ear. I would suggest starting in C Major. With a piano, or any other instrument you are playing, play the scale and sing the notes at the same time – C, D, E, F, G, A, B, C. If you can join with someone else, ask them to play a C on the piano followed by another note in the scale. See if you can work out the note by singing up the scale from C until you reach the note. This may seem slow to start with but remember, you walked before you could run.

Then listen to a song which is in C Major. Using this same process, see if you can work out the notes of the melody and write down what you hear. Once you have written the melody down, try playing it on your instrument and see if it ties up with what you heard.

Once you are happy with songs in C Major, try again with other songs in different keys. Then try using the same process with working out the chords.

Can you get to the stage where you can play in church without needing to use a chord chart? Can you distinguish if something is different on the chord chart from the audio recording?

Each time you complete each of these aural sections, you are joining more pieces together until this section is complete.

Rhythm

This is a different section altogether. Here are some questions to help you with rhythm:

- What time signatures can you play in?
- Can you work out what time signature a song is in when you listen to it?
- Can you keep a steady rhythm when playing your instrument? Record what you play and see how it sounds when you listen to it back.

- A lot of songs are recorded to a click track or metronome, which means the timing is very steady. Try singing along with a song you know well, turn the volume off for a couple of seconds, then turn the volume back up. Keep on trying this, but leave the volume off for longer this time. Turn the volume up again. Are you still in time with the song? The longer you keep the volume off the harder it will be.

Each time you complete these questions you are joining more pieces of the puzzle together.

I would suggest focusing on one of these sections at a time; it may be rhythm, it may be learning your scales. Always ask the question at the end of your practice, what progress have I made? For some of it you might progress quickly, other sections might be slower, but each time you make progress you are joining pieces of the puzzle together until the puzzle is complete. Once you have achieved your goals for each musical section, you have completed the puzzle. That's great, but now you have achieved your goals and completed the puzzle, are you going to set new goals and start a new puzzle?

By working on these sections and completing your goals, it allows you to play with more freedom and therefore you are getting closer to being able to play all that is within you when expressing your worship to God.

Secondary Example – Exercise

I really enjoy exercise and taking on sports challenges, and I am sure many of you will like exercise too, whether it is just for fitness or a sports challenge you want to work towards. Just in the same way as I have used the 'pieces of the puzzle' analogy for music and developing as a musician, you can use this analogy for general exercise to increase fitness or sports challenges too.

Many people who are not into running normally decide they would like to take part in a 5km run for charity. So how do you go about achieving this?

For these challenges you are normally able to download a training plan and this gives you a day-by-day programme to improve your fitness and build up to the 5km run. It may not happen overnight, so within the programme, you can set yourself targets on the way. It may be that you have a ten-week plan and within it you can break it up into sections, setting yourself targets on the way. For example, you might aim to run non-stop:

- 1km after two weeks
- 2km after four weeks
- 3km after six weeks
- 4km after eight weeks

1km could be the edge pieces, 2km could be the buildings, 3km the river and 4km the sky. Each time you complete your two-week target, you have completed another section of the puzzle and once you have finished the 5km run, the puzzle is complete.

Likewise with general exercise, you can break this into sections, for example:

- cardio
- weights
- endurance/stamina
- strength

Working on these different sections, you can set yourself targets and create your own puzzle.

I have used music and worship as an example, but how can you break your limits in something you are trying to achieve? It may be you want to learn a language, it may be a sporting challenge. For what you are trying to achieve, focus on one section or one goal at a time, watch your progression and work towards your target until you have completed it.

Remember, when something is difficult, hard or challenging, with God it is still possible!

Sharing Your Story

I have found it amazing since I started my Breaking Limits ministry how God has opened up so many opportunities for me. I am really keen to share my story wherever I can.

Mark 16:15:

> He said to them, 'Go into the world and preach the gospel to all creation.'

We all have our own story and I would really encourage you to share with others who do not yet believe in God. Although you may not know it yourself at the time, your words may really open up their hearts as God uses you.

Matthew 5:14-16:

> You are the light of the world. A city set on a hill cannot be hidden. Nor do people light a lamp and put it under a basket, but on a stand, and it gives light to all in the house. In the same way, let your light shine before others, so that they may see your good works and give glory to your Father who is in heaven. (ESV UK)

Remember that you are God's vessel and God can speak through you.

2 Timothy 2:20-21:

> In a large house there are articles not only of gold and silver, but also of wood and clay; some are for special purposes and some for common use. Those who cleanse themselves from the latter will be instruments for special purposes, made holy, useful to the Master and prepared to do any good work.

God has a plan for each of us. Jeremiah 29:11 says:

> 'For I know the plans I have for you,' declares the LORD, 'plans to prosper you and not to harm you, plans to give you hope and a future.'

I find it amazing the number of times that situations arise and things seem to fall into place. Ephesians 1:11 says:

> In him we were all chosen, having been predestined according to the plan of him who works out everything in conformity with the purpose of his will ...

I have recently been invited on a ten-day speaking trip to India and for me, although I jumped at it when I was invited, I knew it would take quite a lot of working out as I need a carer; I thought it might be quite complicated to arrange. I told some friends from church that I had been invited, one of whom is from India. He asked whereabouts in India and I told him the name of the town, which I had not heard of before, Vijayawada, and he told me he grew up not far from there and some of his relatives live there. Without even asking, he offered to come with me and give all the help I need. He is a doctor and knows the area and the culture so it could not be more ideal. It is amazing how God places people in our lives!

We all face difficulties or trials at some point but James 1:2-4 says:

> Consider it pure joy, my brothers and sisters, whenever you face trials of many kinds, because you know that the testing of your faith produces perseverance. Let perseverance finish its work so that you may be mature and complete, not lacking anything.

No matter our situation, we always have a reason to praise God because God is:

Our Saviour – John 3:16:

> For God so loved the world that he gave his one and only Son, that whoever believes in him shall not perish but have eternal life.

Our Healer – Isaiah 53:4-5:

> Surely he took up our pain and bore our suffering, yet we considered him punished by God, stricken by him, and afflicted. But he was pierced for our transgressions, he was crushed for our iniquities; the punishment that brought us peace was on him, and by his wounds we are healed.

Our Refuge and Strength – Psalm 46:1:

> God is our refuge and strength, an ever-present help in trouble.

Omnipotent – Matthew 19:26:

> Jesus looked at them and said, 'With man this is impossible, but with God all things are possible.'

Omniscient – Psalm 147:5:

> Great is our Lord, and abundant in power; his understanding is beyond measure. (ESV UK)

Omnipresent – Psalm 139:7-12:

> Where can I go from your Spirit? Where can I flee from your presence? If I go up to the heavens, you are there; if I make my bed in the depths, you are there. If I rise on the wings of the dawn, if I settle on the far side of the sea, even there your hand will guide me, your right hand will hold me fast. If I say, 'Surely the darkness will hide me and the night become night around me,' even the darkness will not be dark to you; the night will shine like the day, for darkness is as light to you.

Sovereign – Isaiah 46:9-10:

> Remember the former things, those of long ago; I am God, and there is no other; I am God, and there is none like me. I make known the end from the beginning, from ancient times, what is still to come. I say, 'My purpose will stand, and I will do all that I please.'

Great – Psalm 145:3:

> Great is the LORD and greatly to be praised, and his greatness is unsearchable. (ESV UK)

So no matter what situation you are facing, remember the scripture from 1 Thessalonians 5:18 because God is our Saviour, our Healer, our Refuge and Strength, Omnipotent, Omniscient, Omnipresent, Sovereign, He is a great God!

> Give thanks in all circumstances; for this is God's will for you in Christ Jesus.

Psalm 145 – A psalm of praise:

> I will exalt you, my God the King;
> I will praise your name for ever and ever.
> Every day I will praise you
> and extol your name for ever and ever.
> Great is the LORD and most worthy of praise;
> his greatness no one can fathom.
> One generation commends your works to another;
> they tell of your mighty acts.
> They speak of the glorious splendour of your majesty –
> and I will meditate on your wonderful works.
> They tell of the power of your awesome works –
> and I will proclaim your great deeds.
> They celebrate your abundant goodness
> and joyfully sing of your righteousness.
> The LORD is gracious and compassionate,
> slow to anger and rich in love.
> The LORD is good to all;
> he has compassion on all he has made.

All your works praise you, Lord;
 your faithful people extol you.
They tell of the glory of your kingdom
 and speak of your might,
so that all people may know of your mighty acts
 and the glorious splendour of your kingdom.
Your kingdom is an everlasting kingdom,
 and your dominion endures through all generations.
The Lord is trustworthy in all he promises
 and faithful in all he does.
The Lord upholds all who fall
 and lifts up all who are bowed down.
The eyes of all look to you,
 and you give them their food at the proper time.
You open your hand
 and satisfy the desires of every living thing.
The Lord is righteous in all his ways
 and faithful in all he does.
The Lord is near to all who call on him,
 to all who call on him in truth.
He fulfils the desires of those who fear him;
 he hears their cry and saves them.
The Lord watches over all who love him,
 but all the wicked he will destroy.
My mouth will speak in praise of the Lord.
 Let every creature praise his holy name
 for ever and ever.

This is just my story of what God has done in my life, but testimonies can be a very powerful tool to share the good news about Jesus. Each of you who are Christians will have your own story and I would certainly encourage you to share this with people.

TV and Media Opportunities

So from starting my ministry in 2016, I have had many speaking opportunities in churches, schools, young offenders' units and with other organisations. This is something I would have never expected to be doing a few years ago. I would have got very nervous if I had to talk in front of people.

One great opportunity I had recently was sharing my story on TBN UK where I was interviewed on their TBN Meets programme. TV and media are such good opportunities as this can reach so many more people than just those I speak to in churches or schools.

For those of you who pray, it would be great if you could pray for me as I continue to share my story, for opportunities to open up and in particular for lots more opportunities in schools. Schools can be hard to get into, but when I get opportunities, I find children react really well, they are very responsive towards me. Having shared my story at a church in Bristol, I was contacted by the BBC Radio Bristol social media team as they saw the advertising for the talk. They asked if they could film a ninety-second clip to share my story to put out on social media. This was great!

BBC Radio Bristol were linking up with a charity called Alive for an appeal show called Britton's Big Night Out, hosted by Emma Britton, a presenter on BBC Radio Bristol. They invited me to play a couple of tracks for the show. There were other really good acts there including people who had made the semi-finals of Britain's Got Talent. So what a surprise and a privilege it was to get invited to play for the show.

How to Become a Christian

—⁓—

Even though I have my own physical disability and challenges, I made my own personal decision to become a Christian at the age of five. I had absolutely no doubt whatsoever about God's existence and I made my own decision and prayed and asked Jesus into my life. Mum explained to me the scripture from John 3:16:

> For God so loved the world that he gave his one and only Son, that whoever believes in him shall not perish but have eternal life.

She then told me that I need to pray and ask Jesus into my heart.

Romans 10:9-10:

> If you declare with your mouth, 'Jesus is Lord,' and believe in your heart that God raised him from the dead, you will be saved. For it is with your heart that you believe and are

justified, and it is with your mouth that you profess your faith and are saved.

Just like I made my own personal decision to become a Christian, you too have the opportunity to make the same decision and invite Jesus into your life. All you need to do is say a simple prayer similar to this:

Dear Lord Jesus, I know that I am a sinner and that I cannot save myself. Thank You for dying on the cross to take away my sins so that I may live eternally with You. I believe You are the Son of God who died for my sins and on the third day You rose from the dead. Thank You for this amazing love you have given me. Jesus, I invite You into my heart to be Lord in my life and be my Saviour. Amen.